How To Reverse Arthritis Naturally

By Dr John Bergman
www.BergmanChiropractic.com

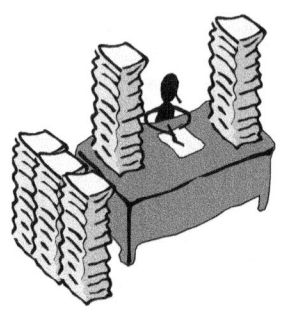

Table of Contents

Disclaimer:

You must not rely on the information in this book and/or video series as an alternative to medical advice from your doctor or other professional healthcare provider.

If you have any specific questions about any medical matter you should consult your doctor or other professional healthcare provider.

If you think you may be suffering from any medical condition you should seek immediate medical attention.

You should never delay seeking medical advice, disregard medical advice, or discontinue medical treatment because of information in this book and/or video series.

Any change in medication, diet, and or exercise should be directed by a qualified health care professional.

Dedicated

This book is dedicated to all the people that have taken charge of their health. To take charge of your own health takes a tremendous amount of courage and responsibility. Today's health care system is based on a symptom drug approach, turning patients into victims that have the bad luck or bad genes to have caught the disease or arthritis. To take charge of your own health in today's health care system really requires you to develop a belief system that health comes from within. To reverse arthritis or any disease requires you to be responsible for your disease as well as your healing, and this takes courage. I practice with the belief system that your body is self-healing, self-regenerating, and self-regulating. Some of my patients have been to 5 or more doctors before coming to my office. What drove them to keep looking for health solutions? When they got a diagnosis from the health "expert", what drove them to look for different solutions? Only when people listen to that inner voice, that voice is the innate intelligence that we all have. When you develop the awareness that there is an innate inborn intelligence and working with this intelligence arthritis can be reversed. The power to heal yourself resides inside of you, lets awaken the power that and watch your joints regenerate!! Throughout this book I will present case studies of actual patients that have made the choices and regenerated their bodies and reversed their arthritis. I have changed their names but their stories and ages are real.

Dr. Bergman

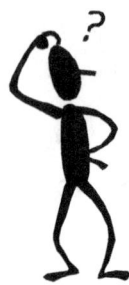

"There are two ways to be fooled. One is to believe what isn't true; the other is to refuse to believe what is true."

— Søren Kierkegaard

Can Arthritis be reversed?

The quote above is vital to ponder when we are confronting a belief system that arthritis is or is not reversible. Arthritis reversal is more about human potential and a change in belief systems. This book will break down the ignorant belief system that has been imposed on the public and doctors alike. This belief system of Arthritis, that it is a progressive and degenerative condition that is inevitable has we age, and the only thing that can be done for arthritis is to make the person comfortable while the joints decay. I have found in over 16 years of practice and thousands of patients that joints are made up of living tissue, ligaments, cartilage, bone, all alive and with the ability to regenerate. The most challenging aspects that I have found in working with patient diagnosed with arthritis is to have them unlearn what the media and doctors have told them.

On doing research for this book I studied several body-building groups. I found one in Japan where the minimum age is 75 years. That's right; you have to be 75 years old to join. A lot of people think that as we age we're supposed to break down, and that's not true. If you don't drive a car, the car is going to last a long time; but if you don't drive a body, it's going to break down early. With human beings, the more we use our body, the longer it works.

I need to explain how I got into researching and practicing arthritis reversal. Picture this: I was a 30-year-old, hard-working single dad. I was jay-walking across the street, and all of a sudden, I was struck by a car. I had both my legs broken, my sternum fractured, my skull fractured, my liver bruised, and my heart bruised. My front teeth were knocked out. I was lucky to be alive, and when I was taken to the hospital,- I got the finest medical care the world has.

Our emergency medical care in this country is the best in the world. They will absolutely take someone that's near dead and save their life. For healthcare the American medical system has a horrible record, but for emergency care, it's incredible.

I was so grateful to the doctors that saved my life. When they suggested knee operations I went agreed; after all, they were the experts. They did the first operation on my knees, and it felt okay; but then they did another operation and it felt worse; and then they did another operation and it felt even worse; and I started to think, "Wait a second. When they're operating, are they putting stuff in or taking stuff out?"

They're taking stuff out. So with these operations, arthroscopic surgery after arthroscopic surgery, I was still hurting, and I was limping. They said, "Of course you're limping. You damaged your cartilage; you damaged your joints. Don't worry about it. We're going to keep you comfortable." They talked about pain medications, and I thought, "Gosh, being drugged." I was so scared that I wouldn't be able to play with my kids. I always wanted to be the dad that I didn't have. My dad died when I was a young kid. I wanted to be there for my kids, and I didn't think I was going to be there. There is nothing more frightening!

So the medical world really wasn't offering me hope. It really wasn't. I was seeing a Chiropractor at the time, and it was interesting, because he was doing adjustments on me while I was in a wheelchair. I don't know if you know this, but if you've ever had two broken legs at one time, you're not mobile. So I'm in the wheelchair, and I'm going in there, and after every operation I'm back in the wheelchair; and wheelchairs are not fun or comfortable. The Chiropractor is adjusting me, and he's saying, "Your body is designed to heal; it's designed to be healthy. Your body can regenerate."

And I said, "No, because I fractured my bones." And he said, "It doesn't matter. Within four or five weeks, your bones are brand new." And I said, "Yeah, but they're operating on my cartilage, my knees, my meniscus." And he says, "Your meniscus can re-grow; it's alive."

And I'm thinking, "Everything this Chiropractor says makes sense and seems to be true." And so at that time I was starting to not believe the medical doctors and their outcome predictions because it was a belief system; it wasn't science. The bleak future health care professionals were predicting for me was based on their beliefs; and they believed that what they said was true. If I had adopted their belief system, I would have a very poor quality of life today.

If I had believed that my body was broken beyond its ability to regenerate, or if I had been sucked into that belief system, my kids would have lost their dad. Thank God I came to the realization that the body is a self-healing, self-regenerating machine. And I truly found out that the surgeons-- God bless them for their surgical skills—were wrong when it came to their perception of health and of human potential. Their perception was wrong. They believed that more surgeries were appropriate and that medications were appropriate.

Disillusioned by the modern symptom-based, mechanistic health care system, I began a quest to find a vitalistic (life) based healthcare model that would help me regain my health. I became a Chiropractor and instructor at Cleveland Chiropractic College in Los Angeles, specializing in Human Dissection Anatomy, Physiology, Biomechanics and multiple Chiropractic techniques. Cleveland Chiropractic College gave me one of the finest educations in the world. I learned about anatomy, physiology, neurology, microbiology and biochemistry. I became skilled in diagnostics and skilled in pathologies; I became one of the finest trained Doctors on the planet

While studying and teaching anatomy and physiology I dissected over 500 human knees, and I got my knees to work. I began to understand the human potential for recovery from damage and disease. Every joint in the body, when we're talking about arthritis, is basically two bones coming together, surrounded by a joint capsule. The bones are covered with cartilage, and this is an amazing structure. Cartilage is alive; meniscuses are alive.

And inside of this beautiful joint here is a super-filtrated blood: synovial fluid. Every time you take a step you rehydrate your knees.

It is vital that you understand how joints work. By swinging the knee, by opening up that knee--and this is just a person walking-- you create a negative pressure and those two joints separate. That negative pressure allows the super-filtrated blood to flow into the joint. So just moving joints, and creating that negative pressure and positive pressure, allows the blood to flow into the joint.

Not only is this vital; it also makes you understand that the health of the joint is dependent upon the health of the blood going into the joint. This is why diabetics, and people with toxic food substances in their bodies, have horrible joints. If the blood is thick, it can't filter in there, and the cartilage doesn't get healthy. So the health of the joints is absolutely dependent on the health of the blood.

This simple formula of; healthy movement + healthy blood + healthy nerve supply = joints can regenerate. Your body is self-healing if you remove what is causing the joints to degenerate then they will regrow healthy.

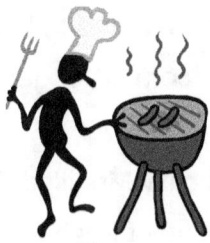

So, is nutrition important when we're talking about arthritis?

Knowing that your body regenerates and in fact you produce over a billion cells per day. The quality of your cells directly effect the quality of your body. Looks like the old saying "you are what you eat" is very literally right!! If you put sick food in your body like; Processed, Genetically Modified, Synthetic, Toxic, then you will be building sick cells and that makes a sick body.

For arthritis as well as all health conditions I recommend 10 vital nutrition changes:

1. Go on a gluten-free, dairy-free diet—because the large proteins in the glutens and the large proteins in the caseins of dairy products, actually thicken up the blood and damage the joints.
2. Eliminate animal proteins; all animal products contain endo-toxins that cause systemic inflammation.

3. Eliminate any polyunsaturated fatty acids like Canola oil, soy oil and soy products, corn oil, vegetable oils (except organic olive oil), safflower oil, etc....
4. Eliminate any Genetically Modified Foods (GMO's)
5. Drink a healthy amount of fresh filtered water (50% of your body weight in ounces every day)
6. Get healthy fats like coconut oil every day
7. Eliminate commercial fast foods
8. Have 80% of your diet raw organic vegetables.
9. Supplement with Algae based omega-3's
10. Take a whole food plant based mineral supplement daily

The 10 nutrition changes are vital to control inflammation. Inflammation is the key to regeneration and destruction, both are vital for healthy joints. There is a difference between systemic inflammation and local inflammation. Both types of inflammation are repair processes; however, systemic inflammation is a response to toxins and will eventually kill you. Systemic inflammation is also a main source of disease. Whereas local inflammation is how discs regenerate and joints heal. The nutrition changes that you must make to reverse arthritis must; clean the blood, eliminate systemic inflammation, control local inflammation, and maximize available nutrients to regenerate your joints.

Case #1 Non-surgical Scoliosis Reduction

Below is an actual patients but I changed her name but her facts and results are real!

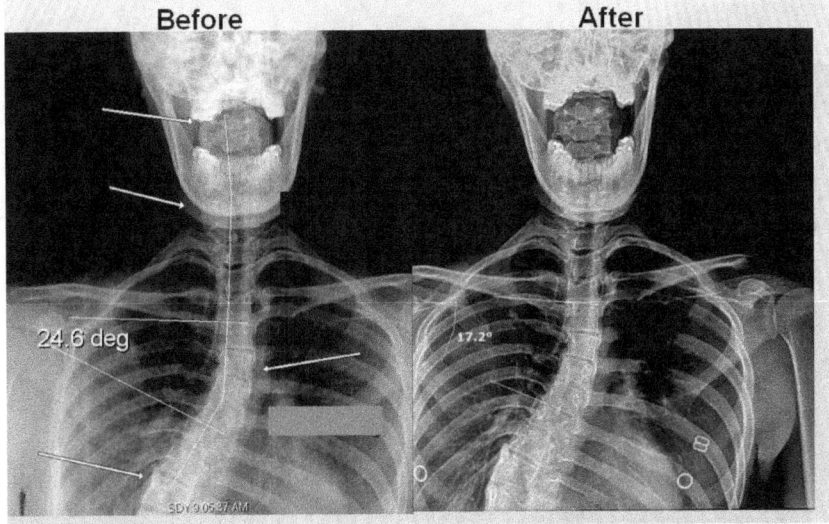

Sue 24 year old woman with scoliosis 30% correction in just 2 years

Before   After

24.6 deg   17.2°

Sue came in to see if I could help her with scoliosis. I was the 4th Doctor she had seen. The advice the other doctors gave went from immediate surgery to her wearing a brace for 22 hours a day. She was desperate for another solution. The vast majority of doctors that treat scoliosis don't know or appreciate that the body can correct the curves of a scoliosis. Sue got these results within the first 6 months of care she had a 30% reduction of her scoliosis and the area that I'm showing is the most challenging area to correct a scoliosis because the thoracic area has 12 ribs on either side designed for protection and not mobility. Corrections in this area are more difficult to achieve. Her care consisted of specific Chiropractic adjustments and supportive exercises only. To get the maximum correction of a scoliosis takes time, healthy nutrition, supportive exercises and corrective Chiropractic adjustments and a change in a belief system of the body's ability to regenerate.

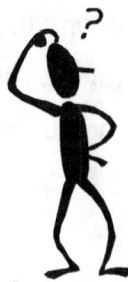

Can the discs of the spine regenerate?

You can't correct arthritis without a healthy nerve supply; so we have to look at the joints of the spine and how these affect the nervous system.

The bones of the spine are called vertebrae. The disc in between is incredibly tough. Imagine this: you know what one layer of fiberglass is like. What if you had 80 inter-connecting rings of fiberglass? Wow, that's tough! In fact, when I was teaching anatomy I would show the students that you could pass a probe (which looks like a thin pencil) right through a bone, but you can't beat it into a disc even with a hammer. Discs are incredibly strong; and they are also 70 percent fluid. Discs are alive and they get their nutrients through movement. Every function of the body is controlled and coordinated by the nervous system. The discs of the spine and the bones of the spine (the vertebrae) protect this vital system. Ninety percent of the nerves that exit the spine don't have any pain fibers. That means they control the body.

How many people get up in the morning and they're stiff-- and then after they move a little bit, the stiffness goes away and they feel okay? That's because there is nerve pressure. Stiffness is like the red light on the dash board of your car, telling you that the nerves that control your body have a problem. If you pinch the nerves to the bladder or the intestines, it will weaken the tissue those nerves supply and lead to bladder infections or intestinal problems (colitis, polyps, diverticulitis, etc).

Discs are under a huge load; for example, the disc at the base of the spine is about the size of a silver dollar. The torso of a 200 pound person stepping off a curb would increase the pressure on that disc about three to four times. There would be 300 to 400 pounds per square inch of pressure on that disc. So blood vessels would be crushed. Because of this natural force loading, the disc has a horrible blood supply, yet the disc gets its nutrients through movement, which increases the nutrient supply.

It's the same as hydrating my knee when I open and close it, or hydrating my elbow when I open and close it. Movement is one of the ways that we can reverse degeneration and arthritis.

We can regenerate discs. I have a couple of surgeons as patients, and one of them happens to be an orthopedic surgeon. He had a really bad neck and his hands were going numb, and he decided he didn't want to get surgery-- because why? Surgery success cases are rare. Some research places the failure rate at up to an 83 percent. That is at best a 17 percent success rate. He didn't want to be a statistic.

When we went over his x-rays, he was aware that he had several discs in his spine that were injured. And he was shocked to learn that discs can regenerate. For this brilliant Doctor to regenerate his discs and recover function of his hands he had to change his belief system that discs can regenerate. This went against his training and education. The reason many Medical Doctors don't know that arthritis is reversible is because of their protocols. The standard medical protocol for neck pain is NSAIDs-- that is ibuprofen®, advil®, motrin®, etc… But those drugs inhibit the building block of cartilage, proteoglycans, which means that the most common initial treatment actually decays the joints. That is why doctors who prescribe those types of medications will not see joint arthritis reversed. Medical schools get a huge amount of funding from the pharmaceutical industry so the standard Medical Doctor's education is skewed towards a drug therapy approach.

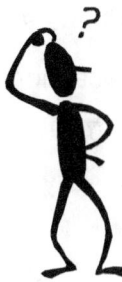

What is Neuropathy?

It's interesting that one of the most brilliant doctors, Dr. William Jacobson, whom I was blessed to have as my mentor, said, "John, to find out what's wrong with the patient you have to do two things: one, you have to ask them; and two, you have to listen." And guess what: it's not as easy as it sounds.

Neuropathy. The most frustrating thing is that doctors look at neuropathy as if it's a disease. But all it means is "nerve problem." Almost everybody has one: carpal tunnel syndrome, or rotator cuff problems, or sciatica-- those are all considered neuropathy.

What's interesting is that when one single nerve is pinched, people will actually say, "Gosh, Doc, I've got this pain that comes right down here." And they will indicate a line that goes from the neck down to the thumb and index finger." And I'll say, "No problem. That's the sixth cervical nerve root. I can fix that." And they say, "How do you know? You haven't even checked it." And I reply, "I can read a map." It's really that simple.

When you see it on a map, you can understand where it comes from. Below is a map of dermatomes which is an area of skin supplied by a specific nerve root

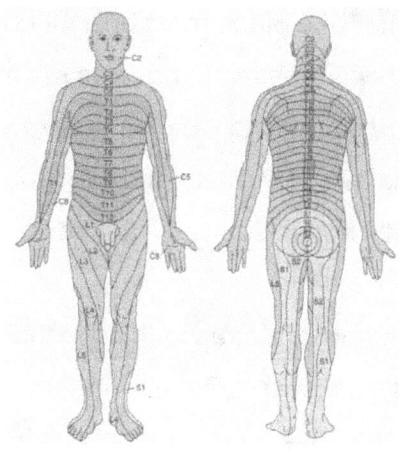

When you look at the sciatic nerve, it's the largest nerve in the body. Any Sciatic symptoms come from a pinched nerve in the low back which is where the sciatic nerve originates. Nerves are always healthy unless there's some kind of neuropathy or pinched nerve in the body. To treat the symptoms of any neuropathy without going after the source of those symptoms will not be effective for restoring health. If you've heard of or have carpal tunnel syndrome, that's a double-crush injury. It begins in the neck and leads to a problem in the wrist.

Have you heard of or do you have rotator cuff or shoulder problems? A rotator cuff injury is a double-crush injury beginning in the neck and leading to shoulder problems. And with all of these conditions, people are getting surgeries that most of the time are not needed. Natural effective alternatives are available for most conditions. The lack of training and lack of awareness of the body's ability to regenerate and reverse arthritis is common in the current health care system.

Some health care professionals say carpal tunnel syndrome is a repetitive motion injury, that's absolutely ridiculous. If it's about repetitive motion, why can some people do the same job and not get the symptom? And why is that 80 percent of the time, carpal tunnel surgery has to be repeated on the other hand? Did they suddenly become left-handed? No. The doctors are missing the *cause* of the carpal tunnel syndrome.

Carpal tunnel syndrome is a double-crush injury; a nerve in the neck is pinched or some of the structures of the neck are compromised, and that leads to a muscle imbalance in the forearm. You have muscles on the back side of the arm called extensors, and muscles on the front side of the arm called flexors– and the strength ratio should be five-to-four flexors vs. extensors. They should be just about equal. But if you look at the average office worker's arm, the muscles on the back side the extensors are flat. And it's usually from a pinched nerve (neuropathy) in the lower neck, and the lower neck supplies the back half of the arm. So it comes from a muscle imbalance-- first a pinched nerve in the neck, then a muscle imbalance of the forearm. Surgery of the wrist for carpal tunnel syndrome is not effective for correcting the source of the problem or the neck. So far at my office we have a 100% success rate of correction of carpal tunnel syndrome because we correct the neck or the source of carpal tunnel syndrome.

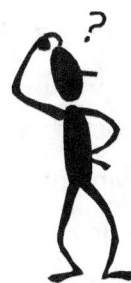

What about herniated discs and stenosis?

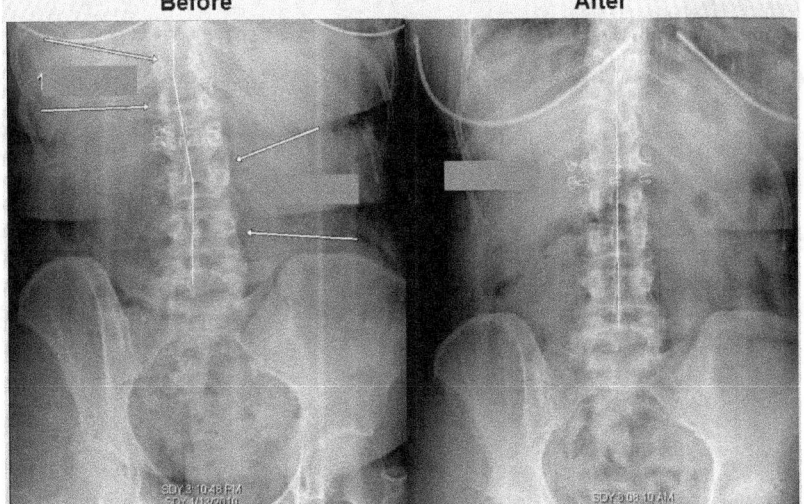

Mary 65 Years Old, Herniated disc on MRI and 20 Years knee pain
Medications: High Blood Pressure, Pain, anti-inflammatories, sleep, anti-acids, Cholesterol, Muscle relaxants

Before	After

Case Study #2 Mary

Mary came to me with a pending surgery for a herniated disc see on an MRI. What most Doctors and few patients don't know is that MRI's are usually done lying on your back. This position will show disc bulges even in healthy people. For an accurate MRI they need to be "weight bearing" that means you need to be seated or standing for the MRI for an accurate reading of the discs. The best way that I have found to assess disc problems is to take standing, weight bearing, stress, digital, x-rays to identify abnormal disc motion.

I addition to Mary's back pain she was taking 8 different medications. Some of the medications she was taking caused horrible side effects and joint pain was one of the side effects of her medications. After 90 days of care her pain was decreased by 80% and her blood pressure and cholesterol went down to normal levels without her medications. Mary's final outcome was repositioning and regeneration of her disc's and her body's functions returned to normal without her medications. That means she is 65 years old drug free and pain free!!

You might have heard of a slipped disc, or a bulging disc, or a herniated disc; it's all the same thing. First, the spine has *abnormal motion*. How does a disc get its nutrients? Through correct motion and correct alignment. So if you have abnormal motion, the disc is not going to have a healthy nutrition supply; and if the disc doesn't have healthy nutrients, the disc will lose its thickness. That causes that hard bone or vertebrae to come down and pinch the nerve, thus causing stenosis or narrowing. To reverse this type of stenosis you have to *regenerate* the disc.

The first sign of a disc injury is stiffness. In ninety percent of the nerves that come off of the spine, there are no pain fibers. So stiffness and tightness is the biggest red flag or warning light that you have beginning nerve damage. That stiffness means that the muscles are locked in, trying to protect the nerves that supply everything. Those nerves supply the kidneys and the pancreas and your immune system; those nerves control and coordinate every function of the body.

Here is the side view of a low back:

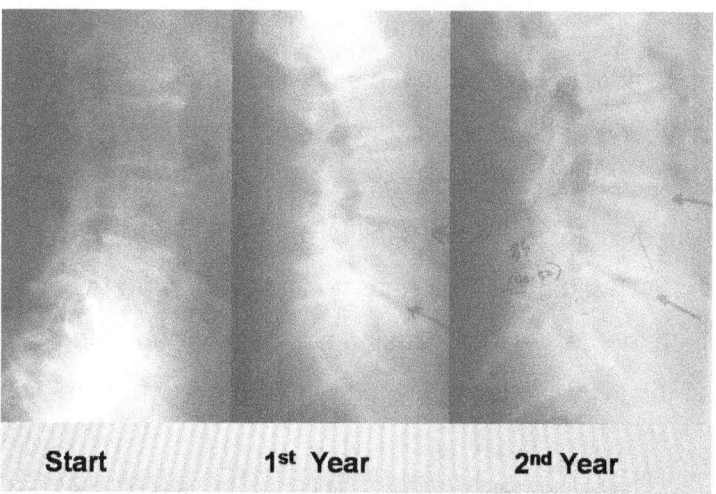

Start   **1st Year**   **2nd Year**

The nerves that come out of the low back supply the back muscles and that is where this patient felt the pain. Those nerves also supply the prostate and the bladder, so prostate issues and bladder issues can also begin with decreased nerve supply from the back.

He came into chiropractic, and in six weeks his symptoms were gone. A year later, you could see the disc regenerating (photo above). Two years later, there was a reversal of stenosis and regeneration of the discs (photo). So the body can reverse arthritis. Discs can re-grow! Most health care professionals don't know that discs can regenerate. Here are two questions to ask a doctor: "Is a disc alive or dead? Do we have dead tissue in our body?"

The answers better be "alive" disc's are alive and "No" there is no dead tissue in the body. Any dead tissue in the body is either recycled or eliminated. So if the disc is alive, does that mean that it needs to take in nutrients, and produce proteins, and eliminate waste products? The answer is—yes.

So if you change that nutrient transfer to the disc, then you change the cellular metabolism of the disc; so that means that you can regenerate discs, right?

Right. Discs can regenerate as long as you can restore movement and realign the spine to a more normal position.

When we're talking about arthritis reversal, the current medical system categorizes certain types of arthritis. The most common type of arthritis is osteoarthritis. Osteoarthritis is also called "Degenerative Disc Disease", or "Degenerative Joint Disease". There is rheumatoid arthritis and the rheumatic diseases, which is where the body is attacking itself; the body is attacking the joints. We're going to talk mainly about osteoarthritis. Osteoarthritis is when either a joint is out of place and it starts to wear out, or it is getting no healthy nutrients and starts to wear out. So it's either a biomechanical or a nutrient problem. Rheumatoid arthritis, or rheumatic disease, is different; it's where the body is actually attacking itself.

The main cause of rheumatic disease and all autoimmune diseases is toxins in the body; and the main sources of these toxins are vaccinations and other neurotoxins from processed and genetically modified foods. The multiple vaccination schedule that is recommended can have a toxic effect and can cause molecular mimicry. There is a great article in the medical journal called The Journal of Autoimmunity:J.Autoimmun, 2000 Feb 14(1) 1-10. It states:

- molecular mimicry is an important factor in autoimmune disease

- …causing many autoimmune diseases including: **diabetes, lupus, scleroderma, rheumatoid arthritis, multiple sclerosis, chronic fatigue syndrome, autism.**

- "Even though the data regarding the relation between vaccination and autoimmune disease is conflicting, some autoimmune phenomena are clearly related to immunization"

- first published in 1985 and since that time substantial evidence has accumulated

When I was a kid, they waited until you were five, and then you got five or six vaccines. Now they inject you with hepatitis B vaccine within 12 hours of being born, and if you go along with the standard vaccination schedule your child, will get 81 shots by the time he is six years old. Vaccines contain foreign animal and viral proteins, along with certain immune system stimulants. As an example of vaccine ingredients, here are the ingredients for just one shot : **Aluminum hydroxide, aluminum phosphate, bovine protein, lactalbumin, hydrolysate, formaldehyde or formalin, glutaraldhyde, monkey kidney tissue, neomycin, 2-phenoxyethanol, polymyxin B, polysorbate 80, yeast protein**

Imagine 80 different vaccines all with different additives, that will produce a tremendous amount of antibodies. Antibodies have two jobs: one job is to find a pathogen or a problem causer, kill it, and then commit suicide.

If you have excess antibodies, we talk about molecular mimicry, and we've known this since 1985. If you get a Hepatitis shot and, you don't have a pathogen, i.e. you don't have Hepatitis B, then those antibodies will attack. If they attack the pancreas, you're going to get diabetes. If they attack the joints, you're going to get rheumatoid arthritis. If they attack the brain, you're going to have autistic disorders or some type of brain damage. One of the reasons autoimmune system disorders are on the rise is the massive over-vaccination of our population. It has only been since 2010 that flu shots are approved for every American from 6 months old every year until death. That experiment has never been done before, and there are no animal models to say that *that* number of medical procedures is effective or safe.

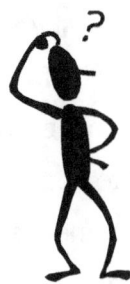

What about autoimmune system disorders Like Rheumatoid arthritis and Multiple sclerosis (MS)?

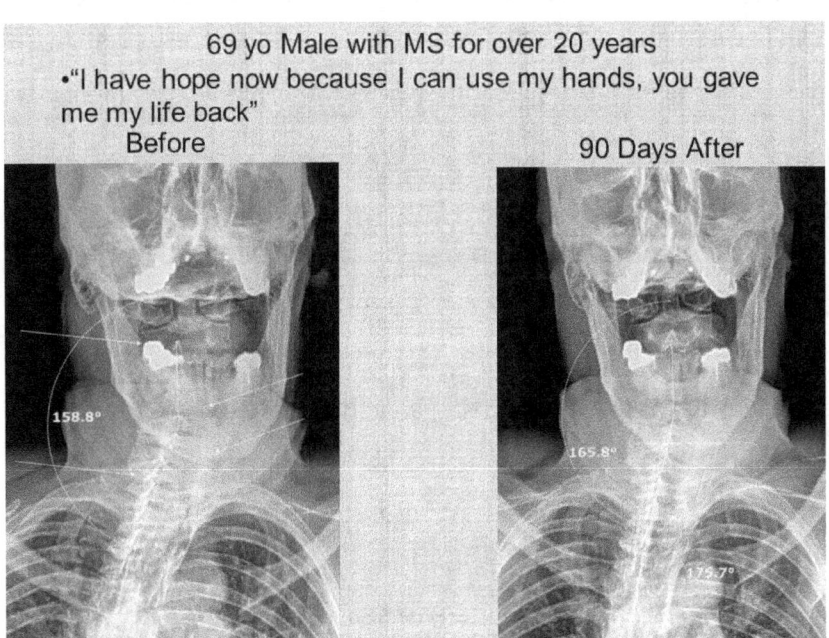

69 yo Male with MS for over 20 years
•"I have hope now because I can use my hands, you gave me my life back"
Before   90 Days After

Case Study #3 Peter

Peter had been diagnosed with Multiple Sclerosis (MS) for 27 years. He came to see me for his back pain. When I first met him his sister had been after him to see me for years and he was not happy, in fact his first words to me were "I'm here to have you fix my back and don't give me any s#*t that you can help with my MS" . My response was "I know I can help with you back pain but I'm pretty sure I can help with your MS". Within 2 weeks his back pain was reduced by 80% and within 8 weeks he started to be able to feel temperature changes with his hands. Within 90 days he was able to tie his shoes!! Just tying your shoes sounds like a small thing, but regaining control of your hands can change a life!

For another example of the Multiple Sclerosis, here is my patient-- let's call her Rebecca. It's interesting because MS is not an arthritic condition, but it *is* an autoimmune disorder. She didn't have a normal curve in her neck, and the only way she was diagnosed with MS is because she started to have tremors; she started to have all sorts of loss of motor control. The doctors did a brain scan and found that she had lesions in the brain, and they said-- get this: I think she was 28 or 30 years old, had two little kids, and they said--"You have multiple sclerosis. You have an incurable disease, and eventually you're going to be in a wheelchair. And you're going to be lucky to see your kids graduate from high school." Think of what that would mean to a young mother-- would that be scary?

If you hold to the belief system, that the nervous system regenerates, and discs regenerate, and bones regenerate, then disease can be reversed! The body is self-regulating and self-healing. Even MS can be reversed if you can find the source. The source of MS is deficiency or toxicity.

So I said to Rebecca: "Let's get pressure off your cervical spine. We'll talk to the doctor who gave you the drugs and let him know you may not need them when you get your body working right." Within 9 months, she had no more symptoms. She went in, had a second brain scan, and the scan found no more lesions. Say it with me: "Cool."

The advice that is typically given for multiple sclerosis: Don't exercise and take steroids to depress the immune system. What do steroids do? They inhibit: they slow down metabolic processes, when actually, with MS, your body is breaking down. To reverse MS you want to build up your body. And the other common advice is: don't exercise. If you exercise, aren't the nerves being stimulated? Yes or yes? Is more oxygen being stimulated? Absolutely! More oxygen and more nerve stimulus-- would that change the metabolic processes of the body? Yes. If you increase metabolic processes could that decrease the demyelization of the nerves that is supposed to be the cause of MS? Yes. These are dangerous questions because this therapy is in direct contrast to the current medical dogma

Another of my patients diagnosed with MS for over 30 years!-- was Bill(not his real name). He comes in. He can't shake hands; his hands are not working well so he shakes hands with his wrist—which he can't bend, and he can't close his hand. He comes in with back pain, a real stoic guy. His understanding is that there is no way that we could help his MS. He just wants his back pain cured and he has heard we are good with correcting back pain. His pain is limiting his passion which is gardening.

According to him, he had been to every expert on the planet, every rheumatologist, every neurologist, everybody. But what do these "experts" do? They don't have the belief system that the body can heal itself. That is the same road block that patients hit when they tell their doctor they want to reverse their arthritis. The average doctor doesn't know arthritis can be reversed so they don't try.

Bill was taking four different blood pressure medications. If your body is breaking down as it is when you have MS, and knowing that the nervous system burns oxygen like a car burns gas, and you have a nervous system disorder, do you think in order to adapt to this disease, or "dis-ease," do you think maybe he would have a higher blood pressure than that of a 21 year old athlete? Yes or yes?

I know enough to realize that there may be different metabolic requirements depending on what the body is dealing with. Like a higher temperature for a viral infection. Using common sense, do you think someone with MS might require different vital signs than someone who doesn't have MS? What does the medical world say? The medical world protocols are based on standards of care and not based on the needs of individual patients.

His medical doctor thought he should have the same blood pressure has everyone else, so they gave him one blood pressure drug. Did that work? No. His body raised the blood pressure higher. How about two blood pressure drugs? No, not good enough. Three? No, not good enough. Four? Okay. When you look at the side effects of the blood pressure drugs, or the unknown effects of mixing four different blood pressure drugs, this could be a disaster. Do blood pressure drugs increase blood flow or decrease blood flow? You got it; they reduce pressure-- that is what they are designed to do. And they decrease blood flow. Remember Bill's hand symptoms? They were swollen and numb and tingling. We got the pressure off Bill's nervous system, and his blood pressure began to normalize. I sent him back to the doctor that prescribed the blood pressure drugs and, sure enough, Bill didn't need them any more. He stopped the drugs and regained about 30% use of his hands within the first three weeks.

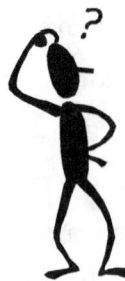

What about autoimmune system disorders Like Rheumatoid arthritis and Fibromyalgia?

Mary (not her real name) 12 years old, came in to my office a few years ago diagnosed with fibromyalgia and rheumatoid arthritis.

The only way to diagnose rheumatoid arthritis is through a blood test that's called "RA positive" and the patient has to have symmetrical joint symptoms. To diagnose fibromyalgia, the patient has to have 18 of 22 tender areas on their body. There is no blood test or x-ray that will show fibromyalgia. Mary's mom wanted me to put her on disability. Think of this: a 12-year-old girl on disability. What's the quality of her life going to be like? Disabled the rest of her life-- it's crazy.

I asked the mom, "Would you mind if I took an x-ray of her?" "No, we've already taken her to the best experts on the planet," was her answer, so I asked again, "Would you mind if I took an x-ray of her?" She let me take the x-ray and what I found was a horrible neck curve. If the neck curve is lost, then the child can either be in chronic pain or there can be a loss of function. So I asked, "Was she born at home or in a hospital?" She was born in a hospital. So we know that it was probably a traumatic birth. "Were you given pitocin at the birth?"I asked the mom. Pitocin is a drug used to stimulate contractions during pregnancy and this can increase trauma to the child."Yes, how did you know?" the mom asked.

Pitocin is a hormone that causes the uterus to contract, so that means that child's head was jamming up against the cervix. So we know there was trauma. "Did the child have multiple ear infections?" "Yes, how did you know?" Because ear infections have to do with the upper cervical ganglia. It supplies the soft palate. After birth trauma, this area is commonly injured, with the soft pallet not working correctly; and the middle ear fills up with fluid, causing pain. This is typically diagnosed incorrectly as an ear infection when it is usually an ear effusion.

So if the child had birth trauma, the soft palate is not going to work, and then the ear is going to fill up with fluid. Eighty-three percent of the time, ear infections are curable with one visit to a chiropractor. Why? Because we take pressure off the neck and that causes the soft palate to work correctly.

Think of this; We know birth trauma; we know ear infections. What do children get for ear infections?

Antibiotics. However, we know that 93 percent of the time the ear infections are sterile, and the American Board of Pediatrics has said "No more antibiotics for ear infections," but doctors are still passing them out. The following is from the journal of clinical infectious diseases 2006:

- Antibiotics have no effect on the viruses found in AOM (Acute Otitis Media) infections, which means that the standard treatment is at best only partially effective for most cases. However, many cases of AOM heal themselves without antibiotic treatment.

- The American Academy of Pediatrics and the American Academy of Family Physicians have therefore recommended avoiding antibiotic treatment in mild AOM cases.

Clinical Infectious Diseases December 1, 2006; 43(11): 1417-1422

So a little girl takes this poisonous mold—the antibiotic, and wipes out the normal gut flora. That causes a leaky gut. The vaccinations (because she's fully vaccinated) and the antibiotics actually bore holes in the intestinal tract, and then large proteins can get in the intestinal tract.

These large proteins-- gluten and caseins-- actually pierce the gut. They're undigested proteins. They also attach to the opiate centers in the brain, starving the brain. This is why kids with attention deficit disorder or certain other neurological disorders have to go on a gluten-free, casein-free diet.

So I see this 12-year-old. I'm just telling you the history of this cute little kid, this darling little angel that I'm not going to put on disability. Can we get her better? Absolutely we can, because we know about the trauma and we can repair the gut and we can get pressure off the nervous system.

And sure enough, we get her to change her diet to, a gluten-free, dairy-free diet to repair the gut, and we get her nervous system working right, and guess what happens? The pain goes away.

Then she went to the rheumatologist, and he must have been Mr. Personality because he did the blood test again-- because something was unusual, because she didn't hurt. And, he said to the mom, "Your daughter's rheumatoid arthritis is in remission."

The mom didn't have more than a high school education; she didn't know what remission was. She came to me and said, "What's wrong with my daughter?" And I said, "She doesn't have the arthritis anymore"

They moved up to the high desert after a few weeks of appointments at our clinic. Then about three weeks after she left care, I got a call from her mom: "Oh, my daughter's so sore. She's screaming. Her legs are so sore. What do I do?" And I asked,

"What was she doing?" The mom said, "I've never seen her run like that. She was playing all day in the park, running around everywhere."

I told the mom to put her into a hot bath. It was common sense: her legs were sore because she had never used them so much. I told the mom not to worry, that her daughter would be fine. And sure enough, the daughter recovered fully with no future diagnoses of any type of arthritis or fibromyalgia.

So when we look at the autoimmune disorders that are causing the different types of arthritis, there is an answer. First fix the body by finding any problems with the immune system. Then fix the gut by eliminating any toxicities or deficiencies. Then fix the nervous system by removing abnormal nerve pressure. Arthritis is mainly a mechanical problem or a problem of deficiency or toxicity.

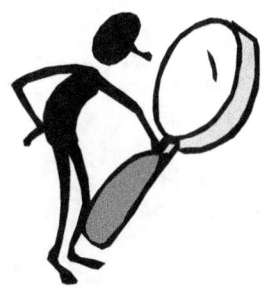

Osteoarthritis or Degenerative Disc Disease or Degenerative Joint Disease

Many doctors and much of the general public think that osteoarthritis is from old age, but that is absolutely, completely untrue. Arthritis is graded one, two, three and four. Grade one means the bone is slightly out of position, but there's no destruction of the disc or bone. Grade two means we're seeing beginning destruction of the disc, and possibly of the bone. Grade three is near fusion, where we're seeing massive destruction of the bone. And grade four is totally fused.

Arthritis: A Mechanical Problem

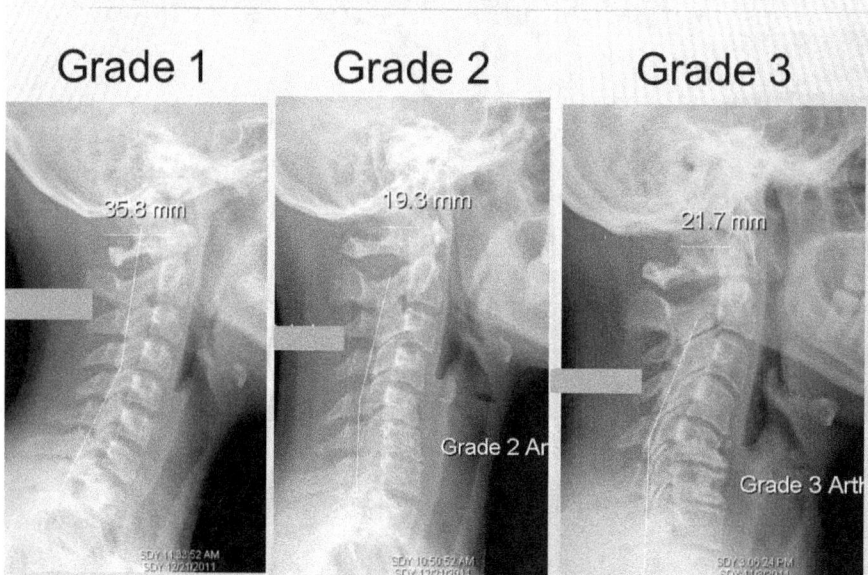

SkypePackage.com / ArthritisReversalSystem.com / Owners-Guide.com

Is arthritis from old age? NO!!!

Arthritis is from trauma!!!

According to:

Managing Low Back Pain, Second Edition, Churchill Livingstone 1988, p 25:

"…degenerative changes do not appear unless the joint has been damaged by trauma. Many elderly joints prove to be just as strong in torsion or compression as younger ones."

"The joints are just as strong. Furthermore, degenerative joints appear to be stiffer than normal, but fail before the healthier ones. So when you have a degenerative joint, it's weaker. It has nothing to do with age. This is a typical mechanical characteristic of scar tissue; it implies scar tissue or injury."

The research above is based on taking joints from cadavers of old people and cadavers of young people.

That means arthritis is a scar tissue. It's damaged. That's all it is. Arthritis doesn't have to happen as we age.

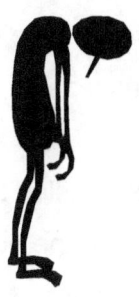

What about arthritis of the neck?

For degeneration of the neck area, look for forward head carriage; because for every one inch that the head is forward, the pressure on the disc below doubles. In a normal head posture when you look at a person from the side view, the ear should line up with the shoulder. If your head is forward two inches, you're talking four to eight times the amount of pressure on those discs. With that much abnormal pressure on the discs of the cervical spine or the neck vertebra, the body is going to increase the tone of the neck muscles to pull the head back in position and reduce that pressure on the discs.

So how do ignorant but well meaning physicians treat a tight muscle? They relax it. Muscle relaxants-- that is one way to relax a muscle. If you're a chiropractor who doesn't check for forward head carriage, you might massage or ultrasound a tight muscle.

Look at why the body is increasing the tone of the muscles. Doctors need to pay attention to the body. If the head is forward, restore the curve in the neck so there are no longer spasms in the body. It makes a lot more sense than trying to drug away the symptoms or doing therapies without understanding the "why" behind the symptoms.

This quote from Voltaire is one of my favorites: "Doctors are men who prescribe medicines of which they know little, for diseases of which they know less, and human beings of which they know nothing."

But it's not a slam on the education of health care professionals; it's a slam on their perception. The revised perception needs to be that *the body is designed for health*. Think of it this way: Pain-- that's not something to cover up. It's a clue to what is going on with the body.

I'm a living example. Two fractured legs, four knee surgeries; I can go jogging or running no problem. I stand up, bend down, turn, twist. Fractured skull, fractured sternum; I have no joint pain. It's incredible.

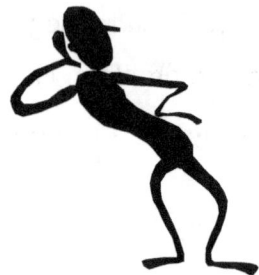

How do we reverse arthritis with inflammation?

Inflammation is how we reverse arthritis. There is a difference between systemic inflammation and local inflammation. Both types of inflammation are repair processes: however, systemic inflammation is a response to toxins and will kill you eventually. Systemic inflammation is also a main source of disease, whereas local inflammation is how discs regenerate and joints heal.

Arthritis can be reversed by causing local inflammation. Local inflammation is how the body heals itself. When I'm adjusting someone, I'm saying, "Yeah, I'm causing inflammation at the level of the disc."

"Inflammation? I heard that's bad." is the usual response I get. No. It's how the body repairs itself. A good explanation of this is:

if you scratch yourself, what color does your skin turn? Red, because that's an increased metabolic process so your body can regenerate itself.

How many times has my arm been scratched? I'm almost 53 years old so, in my life time my arm has been scratched thousands of times. My arm looks good. Because my arm repairs itself, my skin is renewed about every 28 days.

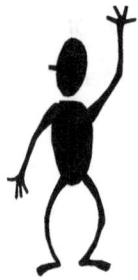

What about anti-inflammatory medications?

Standard drug therapies for inflammation are Tylenol® or NSAIDs, like Mortin®, Ibuprofen®, etc.

Do you know how Tylenol® works in the body? Nobody does; in fact, when you look at the mechanism of action of the main ingredient acetaminophen, it is unknown. That is, we don't know how it works in the body.

One main reason most doctors don't know cartilage can regenerate is that they prescribe drugs that destroy joint cartilage. We're looking at protocols that are completely removed from what normal anatomy and physiology are. The average patient today with joint pain is given a non-steroidal anti-inflammatory for pain relief. Well, that type of drug therapy is going to destroy the joint cartilage. So this therapy will make you comfortable while your body rots. To treat the symptom of pain without correcting the cause of the pain is like putting tape over a warning light on the dash board of your car, that's just dumb.

The following is an article out of the American Journal of Medicine regarding the effects of NSAIDs. They:

- ✖ Decrease cartilage production
- ✖ Inhibits proteoglycan production (the building blocks of cartilage)
- ✖ Causes accelerated bone destruction

      American Journal of Medicine, 1999, Dec.

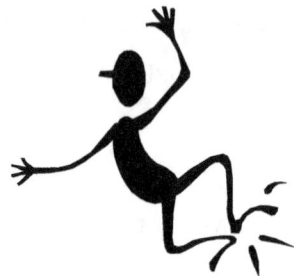

We even use inflammation to correct tendonitis and bursitis!

When correcting bursitis and tendonitis, it is vital to find the cause-- also tennis elbow, golfers elbow, bursitis of the hip. The shoulder, hip and every joint in the body are susceptible to bursitis.

Most movable joints in the body have tendons crossing the joint. Muscles attach to bones by a tendon, and when these tendons cross joints, they are covered by a bursa sac, which is filled with bursa fluid. Bursa fluid is a super filtrate of blood. "Itis" means inflammation, so bursitis is inflammation of the bursa sac from lack of fluid in the bursa sac. This is also the cause of tendonitis. To get tendonitis the bursa sac has to be depleted of fluid this causes friction on the tendon and that causes the tendon to inflame.

I know a lot of doctors who will say that tendonitis is from repetitive motion, and that is just not true. Tendonitis and bursitis are both from lack of blood supply to the joint and/or altered mechanics of that joint. Healthy blood, healthy movement, and healthy nerve supply will equal healthy joints. I have seen thousands of tendonitis and bursitis cases. Every case of shoulder/elbow/wrist/hand bursitis or tendonitis comes from forward head posture and/or subluxations (subluxation is a misaligned bone causing altered nerve flow or altered mechanics) in the neck: and every case of hip/knee/ankle/foot bursitis comes from low back dysfunctions and/or subluxations. For quick relief of bursitis and tendonitis apply moist heat. That's right--I said heat!! That will rush blood supply to the joint and fill the bursa sac with bursa fluid. Once the bursa sac is filled with fluid, that will ease the friction on the tendon and eliminate the tendonitis and bursitis.

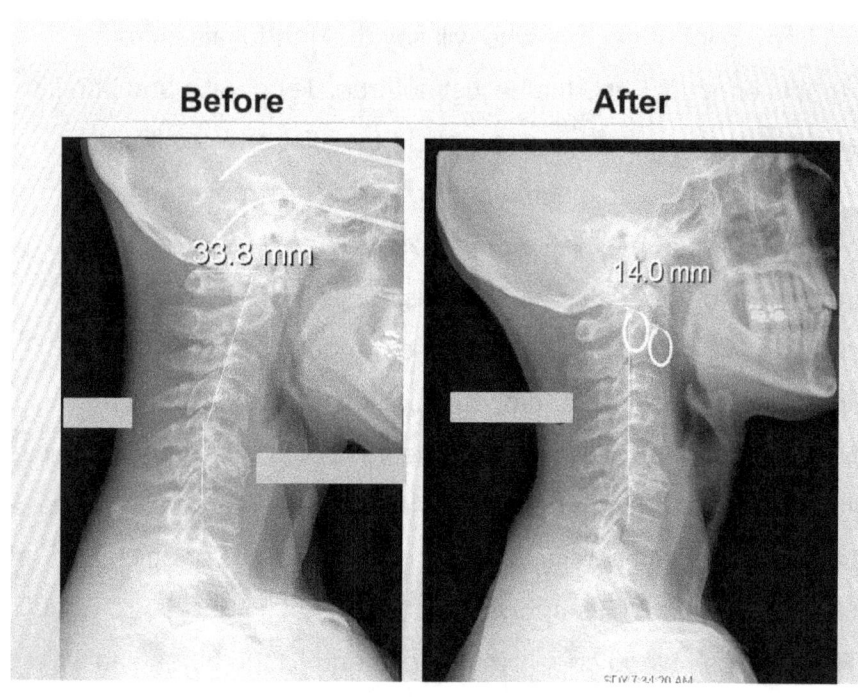

Before	After
33.8 mm	14.0 mm

Case study # 4 Jill

Jill had 38.8mm of forward head carriage and I thought she had a fused disc in her neck from degeneration because I couldn't see a disc space. On her post x-ray not only did her chronic shoulder and wrist pain, vanish but her forward head carriage reduce to 14 mm and her disc began regeneration. This was a good lesson for me that even though I couldn't see a disc the body is smarter than me and regeneration can occur even when I didn't think it could!

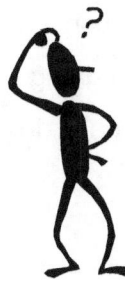

What is the best type of heat?

Local moist heat is the best. A jacuzzi or sauna would not be good or effective for causing a local inflammatory response, which is healing for joints. Sauna's and Jacuzzis are good for various conditions; however, when we are focused on rebuilding joints, you want local moist heat, not heating up the whole body.

The effect you want is to increase the blood pressure at the joint, and that is what local moist heat does. This, in turn, increases the metabolic processes. That means by applying local moist heat, you will increase the production of synovial fluid and increase the production of bursa fluid, and this heat will also increase all of the cells of your body to do their jobs.

Regeneration only occurs at the cellular level and the following is how regeneration occurs. This process goes on whether you want it to or not; your body is constantly regenerating and constantly breaking down. I'm going to show you how to build your body up faster than it breaks down, and this is how arthritis is reversed.

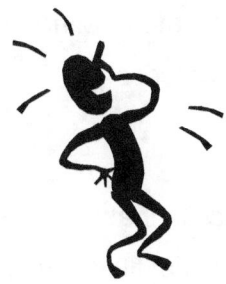

Here – are – a - few – of – my - Favorite - Cells!!!
(Sing this to the Sound of Music theme)

Macrophages - Chondrocytes – Osteoblasts and Osteoclasts

Macro Phages

Called "Big Eaters," these cells eat up abnormally placed proteins. This means that minor tears of ligaments, meniscus or broken blood vessels all get eaten up, and the materials get recycled back into the system to be reutilized to regenerate new tissue. This scavenger or clean-up process is vital to tissue regeneration. Once a joint has been damaged, you have to break down the scar tissue and eliminate the broken and damaged cells. Just think of a bruise that is from breaking blood vessels due to a trauma. The macro phages get to work and break those blood proteins down, cleaning up the site of injury so new tissue can be laid down or regenerated. Minor tears or injuries can be repaired naturally by this process.

Chondrocytes

Chondrocytes are the cells that regenerate cartilage. Cartilage gets its nutrients from synovial fluid. Synovial fluid is a super filtrate of blood, so it is vital that you have healthy blood to stimulate cartilage production. I have seen thousands of patients who have been told by their doctors that their joints are "bone on bone" when it was just not true! If a joint can bend, even if bending a joint is painful, that joint is NOT bone on bone. If a joint can't bend, then it may be bone on bone, and it will not regenerate. A good test of a joint is to apply moist heat for a few minutes. If this increases the range of motion, or if this decreases pain, then we can rebuild the joint. The moist heat fills the structures of the joint like the joint capsule and fills the bursa sacs with fluid. If just filling the joint structures cause greater range of motion then the joint will heal if we can get better blood supply to the joint. That will hydrate the cartilage and help regenerate the cartilage. One of the main building materials for cartilage is proteoglycans.

The major reason why most doctors don't see cartilage regenerated is the therapies that are suggested when a joint hurts. The most common therapy is to prescribe medications at the first sign of joint pain. The most common prescription is Tylenol® or some type of NSAID's like Mortin®, Ibuprofen®, etc.. Those drugs inhibit the building blocks of cartilage or proteoglycans. The purpose of those drugs is to decrease local inflammation. Local inflammation is actually a repair process. That is why it is essential to apply moist heat to increase the blood supply and increase cellular activity in order to regenerate cartilage and restore the joint. Healthy joint *movement* is also essential to regenerate cartilage. To have healthy joint movement you need healthy nerve supply to the joint and proper joint alignment.

Cartilage is a cushion. As an example, let's look at the knee. Nearly all the joints of the body function similarly to the knee. This process with slight variations will work for hips, shoulders, fingers, elbows, wrists, feet, ankles, etc.

The knee is a great example because it is the largest joint of the body and it is commonly injured. I have a lot of experience with rehabilitating knees, because I broke my right knee twice and my left knee once, and I have had four knee operations. Of those four operations, only one of them helped restore proper biomechanics.

That is the main driving force behind my development of joint regeneration. When you are walking, the knee gets compressed because you have weight on it; and when you swing the knee during walking, there is a negative pressure causing fluid to flow into the joint and providing the cartilage with nutrients. To regenerate the knee, you have to decompress the joint without *compressing* the joint. This sounds complicated, but just think of a kid dangling his legs over the edge of a table. That is one of the best exercises to regenerate cartilage.

Depending on any limitations, the patient can have a 3lb to 8lb ankle weight to increase the negative pressure on the knee joint. This will also strain the ligaments, making them stronger as well as regenerating cartilage.

This could be a dangerous exercise for some because you don't want to lift the leg too high; that could drive the knee cap or patella into the joint, so just dangle. If you can apply moist heat when dangling the legs and using the ankle weights … Wow! What an effect you will get. I demonstrate this technique on my video series that goes along with this book.

http://0s4.com/r/LHOZK0

Osteoblasts and Osteoclasts

These amazing cells lay down bone and tear bone up. You need this remodeling process to be going on constantly as long as you are alive.

Your entire body is replaced at an amazing rate.

- ✓ Bones are replaced every 8 to 11 months
- ✓ The lining in stomach and intestine every 4 days
- ✓ The Gums are replaced every 2 weeks
- ✓ The Skin replaced every 4 weeks
- ✓ The Liver replaced every 6 weeks
- ✓ The Lining of blood vessels replaced every 6 months

This constant renewability of your body is a fact that is missed and not appreciated by most doctors or by most of the public today. Every book I write, and every lecture I have given over the last 15 years, is to change people's perception and emphasize the true beauty and amazing nature of our human body.

But let's also look at the *mental* barriers to healing. Bones are renewed; bone spurs are a protective mechanism to protect an unstable joint; discs can regenerate; cartilage can re-grow; bones can become stronger at any age; and the biggest truth is that "bone spurs can be reabsorbed". Sometimes society is not ready for the truth—for example, the idea that the world was round scared a lot of people. Whether you believe in gravity or not, you are still affected by it. The joints of the human body are dynamically changing, whether you know about it or not.

I'm going to tell you how to use those processes to generate healthy joints instead of regenerating unhealthy joints. The fact is: your joints a year from now will be different than the joints you have today. I want you to choose a *healthier version of you*. When we talk about osteoclasts and osteoblasts you have to own the fact that these cells are working all the time. There is a theory called Wolff's Law –it is basically that bone is laid down where needed and resorbed where not needed. When remodeling joints or reversing arthritis, we stimulate the resorption of bone and stimulate the laying down of healthy bone tissue.

Osteoporosis, or a thinning of bone, is mainly from an acidic environment. A good way to look at this is: if your blood is acidic from a toxic life style like fast food, smoking cigarettes, etc. Your body, in order to maintain a health blood PH, will go to the bone bank and with withdraw calcium to alkalinize the blood. This is why, in order to have healthy bones and healthy joints you have to have a healthy diet. In order to stimulate osteoblasts, you have to strain the bones--just minor exercise will stimulate bone production. In fact, many gyms now have vibration plates that you can stand on to stimulate bone production. A simple small trampoline like a rebounder will also stimulate bone production.

There are drugs that are commonly prescribed to thicken bone such as Fosamax®, which is a class of drugs called bisphosphonates. The problem with these drugs is that they stop the osteoblast and the osteoclast activity. This makes the bone appear thicker on a bone densitometer but studies show that the bone is actually weaker.

"The long-term use of osteoporosis drugs known as bisphosphonates can actually weaken bones by impairing their ability to heal, leading to fractures…", according to a study from *New York-Presbyterian Hospital/Weill Cornell Medical Center*

If you are taking that type of drug, educate the doctor that prescribed them regarding the dangers; or find another doctor who is aware of the dangers. Other life style choices that will cause weakening of the bones are : high dairy consumption (that's right; dairy weakens bone), a diet high in animal proteins, anti-acid medications, bisphosphonate drugs, and many other medications.

Diets that strengthen bones are high in dark green leafy vegetables and low in animal products. We have been trained since we were kids to look at the food groups of meat and dairy as being good for us, but diets high in animal products actually weaken bones. And as we age we produce less acid in our stomachs. Stomach acid is essential to break down proteins to amino acids and vital to absorb calcium. With less stomach acid available you may have less calcium available for new bones. To rebuild bones quickly, I recommend juicing dark green veggies in order to get good raw materials to build healthy bones. Also, an essential vitamin is vitamin D-3. The sun is the best source if you live in an area that has good sunlight. For healthy bone, I recommend healthy supplementation of vitamin D-3 and healthy sunlight exposure. There are now many books are out there breaking the myth that sunlight is bad for you. The sun is extremely beneficial. Not so much that you burn your skin but not too little either. Your best amount of sunlight should be directed by a doctor who understands the benefits of the sun.

Understanding how to use Macrophages, Chondrocytes, and Osteoblasts and Osteoclasts is the key to regenerating healthy joints.

Avoid any pharmaceutical anti-inflammatories like Tylenol®, Mortin®, Ibuprofen®, etc… because they destroy the building blocks of cartilage. For pain relief take a good omega-3, preferably algae based. In fact omega-3's have been shown to cause better pain relief than pharmaceutical anti-inflammatories-- without destroying the joints.

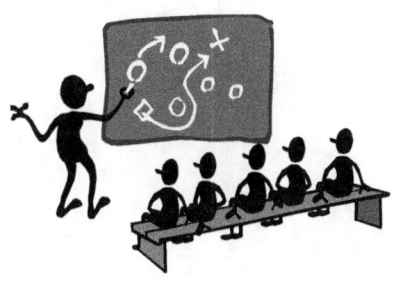

For a bursitis recap:

Correcting the cause of the bursitis problem requires 3 steps:

1. Correct the forward head posture or the low back problem by seeing a corrective Chiropractor.

2. Clean the blood by getting plenty of soluble fibers found in vegetable juice. This will supply natural anti-inflammatories and allow a healthy blood supply. Also eliminate inflammatory causing foods like gluten (grains) and caseins (dairy) and eliminate animal products. These have endotoxins and will also cause inflammation. Drink plenty of fresh spring water-- about 50% of your body weight in ounces daily. A 200 lb man needs at least 100 oz of water per day.

3. Check for muscle imbalances to every joint involved. This requires a skilled Doctor and very simple exercises.

The following are instructions for skilled doctors regarding where to check: For the shoulder, check the Pectoralis Major. For the elbow and wrist, check for weak extensor muscles. For hip or knee problems, check for patellar tracking. For ankle and foot problems, check for calf tightness. I have videos on how to perform these tests.

Upper extremity:

http://0s4.com/r/UPPER

Lower extremity:

http://0s4.com/r/LOWER

You know when you see, because I read all the time, you see these quotes and you just get goose bumps? "We have not lost faith, but we have transferred it from God to the medical profession." George Bernard Shaw

What you need to have healthy joints, and to reverse arthritis and degeneration, is healthy blood. You need healthy movement, because joints need movement and they need correct movement. That's what I do. I restore the nerve supply and blood supply and movement. You need a healthy body, and don't poison yourself. It's really that simple.

This is what we have to do. We don't have to change the medical system; we have to change our perception. If you say, "My joints hurt because I'm over 30," you're wrong. Your joints are only about a year old, no matter your actual age; they're constantly regenerating. Human potential is where I want you to focus. That is true health.

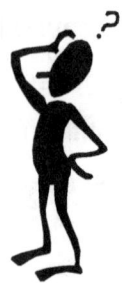

What about the function of blood?

The function of blood. One of the main causes of arthritic changes is the fact that people are lowering their blood pressure when they don't need to. They're chemically altering blood pressure to maintain it at some arbitrary level. If high blood pressure was a danger, there would be warnings on gym equipment: "Goodness gracious, don't lift that weight; your blood pressure will go up!!"

What happens when weightlifters lift weights? What color does their face change to? Red Ask yourself why. It is because to lift great weights, your blood pressure has to increase. When you are straining, the blood pressure can be 400/200. Your body is designed to handle higher blood pressures. I encourage you to check out my book "How to correct High Blood Pressure without

Medications" I have detailed information on how the body regulates itself and how to restore normal blood pressure levels.

So it's not high blood pressure that causes disease. If the body is damaged, the blood pressure increases to adapt to the damage. A prolonged discussion about blood pressure is beyond the scope of this book. Look to the cause of why your blood pressure has been diagnosed as "high". It is the cause of "High Blood Pressure" that needs to be changed. To lower blood pressure with a drug and without treating the cause of why the blood pressure is high will lead to disaster.

Your blood pressure will constantly change depending on your body's requirements. This increase or decrease in blood pressure is an adaptation to keep a healthy supply of oxygen and other nutrients flowing to your many body systems. Responsible doctors will look to the *source* of why the blood pressure is high. Perhaps you have clogged arteries or arterial damage. If so, a good solution would be to give you soluble fibers, which can clean your arteries. Let's change your diet and nutrition. Let's change the toxicity that's causing that arterial damage. Then your blood pressure will decrease naturally." Does that make more sense? Yes or yes?

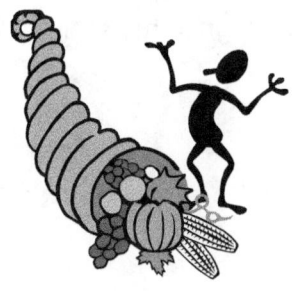

The nutritional aspect of arthritis reversal

To have healthy joints, you have to clean the arteries. To clean the arteries, you have to have soluble fiber. Vegetable juicing is vital for recovery. The best juicer is a slow speed masticating type. My personal favorite is an Omega VRT-350. To start my patients off, I usually recommend 30 – 60 oz per day. My favorite blend is below, and if you store it in mason jars in your refrigerator, it should stay fresh for about 3 days. It produces 20, 16oz mason jars of juice.

Veggie Juice Recipe

Three 3lb bags of Apples (Malic acid to clean the arteries)

Two 5 lb bags of Carrots(good for the lungs)

Six bundles of Spinach(great for protein)

Three bundles of Celery(high in minerals)

Special add-ons for juice:

Garlic for colds/flues

Ginger for stomach issues

Kale for strong immune system and iron

Bell peppers for extra vit. C

Strawberries (organic only)

Beets + Beet Greens (Great for cleaning arteries)

More food suggestions include eliminating meat and all animal products for at least 90 days. Animal products have endotoxins. These cause systemic inflammation and will delay joint repair.

Respect the body, realizing the body is designed to be healthy; it makes so much more sense.

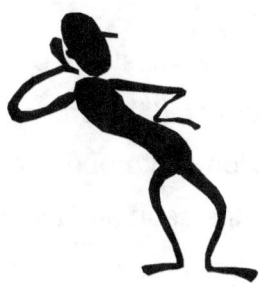

How important is healthy nerve supply and good joint alignment?

"Subluxation" is a term for a bone that is slightly misaligned from it's normal position. A subluxated vertebra is a vertebra that has lost its normal position in relation to the vertebra above and below. Bones of the shoulder, elbow, wrist, hand, hip, knee, leg, and foot can also become subluxated. If there is a subluxation present, this can alter the movement of the joints. It can even alter the nerve supply, and if it is affecting the nervous system, it can change the tone of the structures surrounding the joints. You need a healthy nerve supply to have healthy joints.

For joint pain or degeneration of the shoulder, arm, hand, and fingers, it is vital you get checked for forward head carriage and subluxations of the neck and thoracic areas. For joint pain or degeneration of the hip, knee, leg, or foot, look for subluxations of the low back. Also look for an unstable pelvis and proper foot biomechanics. I have corrected hundreds of knee problems by restoring good calf function and proper foot biomechanics. The area of pain may not be the source of the problem. It is vital that your doctor looks at the entire body's function and not just the site of the symptom. Keep asking that vital question: "Why"?The quality of your life depends on the quality of the questions you ask.

How important is exercise?

You need exercise in order to have healthy joints and reverse any damage. I provide many exercises in the video that accompanies this book. Most of them are ligamentous. That means they are designed to rehabilitate the joints and support the ligaments. Ligaments hold the bone to bone so strong ligaments give you strong joints.

http://0s4.com/r/EXERCI

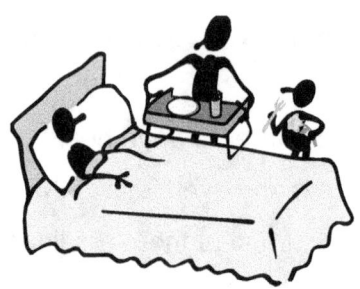

How important is sleep to reversing arthritis?

You have two parts of your autonomic nervous system. One part keeps you alive under stressand it's called the Sympathetic Nervous System (SNS) or the "fight or flight system". The other half of your autonomic system is the Parasympathetic Nervous System (PNS) or the "rest, digest and repair system". You can imagine how important your PSN is in rebuilding joints and reversing arthritis. You live on this planet and you have certain rules you have to live by-- gravity is one of the rules.

There are also circadian rhythms that will affect you. At night between 11pm and 1am is when your PSN is most active. You must have deep sleep at that time. Deep sleep is described as R.E.M. or Rapid Eye Movement. Erratic sleep patterns, and watching TV before bed, as well as a number of different activities, can interrupt R.E.M. sleep. If you don't get healthy sleep, you will not be able to regenerate a healthy body.

If you suffer from insomnia that can be cured within 21 days. Here is a link to my video detailing how to get deep sleep.

http://0s4.com/r/SLEEP

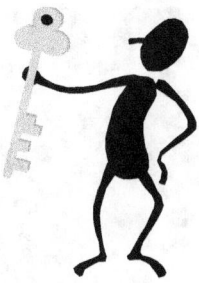

Why is Prayer and Meditation important in reversing arthritis?

Every study that I have seen shows an increase of tissue repair and immune system function when there is a positive mental attitude. The current state of our understanding of anatomy and physiology, from a quantum physics point of view, is that we truly are more energy than matter. With that understanding, and armed with the knowledge that Muslims, Jews, and Christians all agree we are made in the image and likeness of God, daily prayer and meditation is a vital component to any healing.

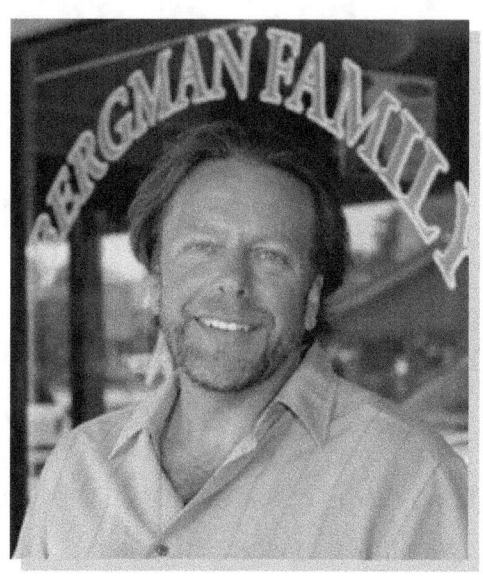

In conclusion, follow the simple formulas in this book and you will achieve optimal health. Health is your natural state! Don't accept decay and degeneration as normal! Your body is self-healing and self-regulating. Next time you walk by a mirror, smile== you are an amazing person!!

Yours in Health

Dr. John Bergman

I am creating a phenomenal tool to give you a step-by-step guide on how to reverse arthritis naturally. It will consist of several videos, manuals and emails specific to reversing your arthritis and getting you back to a pain free life.

For more information, go to ArthritisReversalSystem.com.

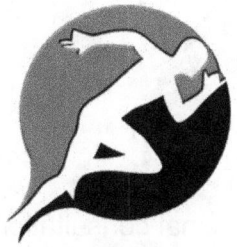

Arthritis Reversal System

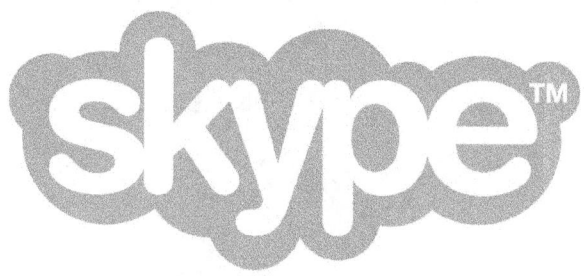

If you would like a personal consultation with me, but can't make it to Southern California, go to SkypePackage.com and we can meet online!

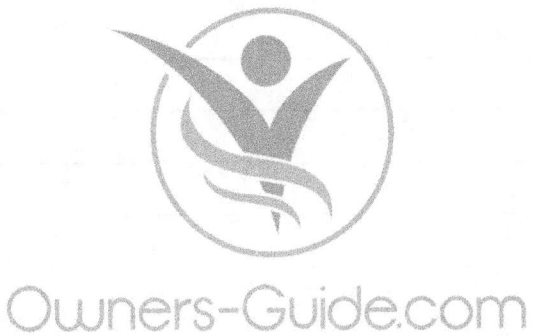

Owners-Guide.com

You can also join our online community at Owners-Guide.com. Enjoy discounts on books, special events, a private FaceBook group and more!

NOTES

_____

_____

_____

_____

_____

_____

_____

_____

_____

_____

_____

_____

_____

_____

_____

_____

_____

_____

_____

NOTES

_____

_____

_____

_____

_____

_____

_____

_____

_____

_____

_____

_____

_____

_____

_____

_____

_____

_____

_____

_____

NOTES

_____

_____

_____

_____

_____

_____

_____

_____

_____

_____

_____

_____

_____

_____

_____

_____

_____

_____

_____

_____

_____

NOTES

_____

_____

_____

_____

_____

_____

_____

_____

_____

_____

_____

_____

_____

_____

_____

_____

_____

_____

_____

_____

_____

NOTES

_____

_____

_____

_____

_____

_____

_____

_____

_____

_____

_____

_____

_____

_____

_____

_____

_____

_____

_____

_____

NOTES

_____

_____

_____

_____

_____

_____

_____

_____

_____

_____

_____

_____

_____

_____

_____

_____

_____

_____

_____

NOTES

NOTES

_____

_____

_____

_____

_____

_____

_____

_____

_____

_____

_____

_____

_____

_____

_____

_____

_____

_____

NOTES

_____

_____

_____

_____

_____

_____

_____

_____

_____

_____

_____

_____

_____

_____

_____

_____

_____

_____

_____

_____

NOTES

_____

_____

_____

_____

_____

_____

_____

_____

_____

_____

_____

_____

_____

_____

_____

_____

_____

_____

_____

www.ingramcontent.com/pod-product-compliance
Lightning Source LLC
Chambersburg PA
CBHW070546290526
45790CB00002B/596